HEADSCARVES, HEADWRAPS & MORE

How to Look Fabulous in 60 seconds with Easy Head Wrap Tying Techniques

Kaye Nutman

HEADSCARVES, HEADWRAPS & MORE

Disclaimer

This book is designed to provide information on Headscarf and Head Wrap tying. This information is provided and sold with the knowledge that the publisher and author do not offer any medical or other advice. This book has not been created to be specific to any individual people or organisations, situation or needs. Every effort has been made to make this book as accurate as possible; however, there may be typographical and/or content errors. This book should serve as a general guide only, and not as the ultimate source of subject information.

Most of these photos were taken by the author, who does not profess to be a professional photographer of any kind. She wishes she could have afforded to hire one, but the results you see here were done to the best of her ability, and do give a good idea of the results you can achieve.

This book may contain slight variations to the print version based on the formatting needs of eBooks.

Publisher: OggyTheOg

Testimonials

"Kaye has volunteered her services at Cabrini Hospital in Melbourne, Victoria for over 6 years, 4 of which have been dedicated to establishing the hospitals free wig service.

Hair loss during treatment can be a confronting time and the patient's first exposure to the wig room can be an emotional one. Cabrini's wig room provides our patients with much more than wigs. Head coverings and scarves are an essential resource for our patients during this time. The most common question asked is "how do I tie a head scarf?'. Kaye's experience and approach helps make the process an easy and pleasant one.

This book will bring a much needed resource to our patients and to many others. Her love for helping others to feel good about themselves shows in her dedication and passion in this book.

I want to thank her for her dedication to help others."

Vicki Durston

Breast Cancer Service Coordinator

Cabrini Health

Brightways – Breast Cancer Service

"Through her sensitive awareness to a need, Kaye Nutman has written 'Headscarves, Headwraps & More'. In this book, she offers a practical and well-illustrated guide to creating various headgear. She ably shows, explains and guides the reader through to the final result. Kaye has worked for several years in a hospital setting, supporting clients through their various medical treatments. She has written many Biographies and engaging children's books and demonstrates a keen eye for colour, design and flair. I am one of a team of ladies, who has worked with Kaye in the 'Wigroom' –a hospital support facility. Here we offer both wigs and headwear to clients wishing to enhance their appearance. My background as an Educational Psychologist has reinforced in me, the importance that self-nurturing has on one's general wellbeing and in dealing with the many life challenges we face. I know this book will be of great service to you or your loved ones who wish to extend their headwear repertoire."

Sue Perriman

Educational Psychologist and Wig Room Volunteer

Melbourne, Australia

Kaye's volunteering experience in Cabrini's Wig Room in Brighton Victoria was the catalyst for her book. I have known Kaye as a fellow volunteer since the beginning of the enterprise, and have seen how her book has evolved. We have spoken enthusiastically and endlessly about scarves, their qualities and where Kaye sources them. She found op shops and general shops to be a good source of inexpensive ones with the occasional expensive one that she couldn't resist! I believe that Kaye's book will be a valuable addition for the clientele we see in the Wig Room, and for anyone else who loves scarves and wearing them."

Ann Michod

Wig Room Volunteer

Cabrini Hospital, Brighton

"Kaye fell in love with headwear from the moment we started up the "Wigroom". She has a knack for being creative and a desire to help clients feel great when they need it most.

Her background in teaching has certainly helped with the process involved in getting this wonderful book together. I applaud her efforts and am sure many people will find her book a great resource."

Robyn Taylor. R.N.

Volunteer/Wigroom,

Cabrini Health.

Dedication

To all women who **_Love_** them, **_Use_** them, or **_Need_** them!

Headscarves, Headwraps & More

1. Acknowledgements

To my husband, Andrew, and son, Alex - Thank you for your patience with me in following this passion. From - (Sigh) "Oh no, not another Op Shop" when I spotted a charity shop; always on the lookout for unique scarves - To, "Mum I've shown you how to do this before!" when asked - yet again - for some bit of computer knowledge... well, boys, you did it anyway. Thank you lovely guys; I truly appreciated your help.

I would like to acknowledge the support of my colleagues and hospital staff at the 'Wig Room' (Day Oncology), Cabrini Hospital, Brighton, where I volunteer. Since a colleague said - "you enjoy tying headscarves so much - you should write a book" - the idea refused to bubble back down, and here it is, so... Thank You!

My head scarf models - Michelle, Brigid, Casey, Pat and Anne - gave some fun packed days of their time and enthusiasm, for little reward other than a cuppa and a few giggles. I really enjoyed those sessions, your willingness, inventiveness and encouragement. You are superb girls. A huge thank you!

Thank you to Kathy at Munchkin Mannequins who provided me with 'Eddie' (and six of her mannequin heads take pride of place each Tuesday the Wig Room is open).

Thanks go out wholeheartedly to those who donated scarves for use in my book – most abundantly, Jennifer Fraser and Kerry Crossingham.

To *Wrapunzel,* who allowed me to use their photo of the Volumisers in the Second section, and whose blog inspired me.

Finally, many thanks go to the talented illustrator, **ANNA MOSS**, who was a joy to work with. Her CAD designs were drawn and tweaked as she toiled away on the other side of the world, whilst I slept. It was so exciting to wake up to something new in my inbox each day.

Table of Contents

2. A Word from the Author

Like to know how to wrap attention grabbing (or discrete) headwraps? Do you look in the mirror and despair at the state of your hair? Clueless about how to tie headwraps that stay put and make a statement?

This book will teach you how to tie compliment attracting headwraps in no time at all! It can be so easy. The styles look amazing in less time than it would take you to curl (or straighten) your hair. They can boost your look in seconds!

Imagine walking out the door, feeling great; confident, covered and chic!

After years of practice and research, showing others how to tie headwraps - hands on, I can now share these wonderful tying techniques with you.

So *Welcome* to the wonderful world of scarf and head wrap tying. The following pages have 26+ wonderful ideas for tying head wraps and scarves. Each design has clear instructions; a full page CAD (Computer Aided Design) illustration, and a photo (or two) of real women - or 'Eddie' the mannequin. This gives you *the best* chance of easily replicating the designs on your own head. There's a BONUS section too.

Because of my volunteer position, I began writing this book with chemo patients in mind; but these amazing designs are so useful to *everyone* who wants to wrap.

Experiencing hair loss due to chemotherapy, or alopecia? How self-assured and amazing you will feel wearing a carefully chosen scarf.

Perhaps you wear a headscarf for religious reasons or modesty.

Maybe you just love fashion – well, wow, what a statement a headscarf can make!

There may be a bad hair day, a breezy morning at the beach, dog walking, a cruise or a party - any number of reasons... you tell me (*please*... write to me!).

My website: - www.kayenutman-writer.com

Why I wrote this book

I volunteer in a Wig Room.

What's that, you may say?

It is a hospital initiative to provide *free* wigs and headwear to its chemotherapy patients, and extends to *anyone* undergoing chemo in Bayside and the area served by the hospital. Over the four years it has been open, one of the frequently asked questions after wig fitting is… "How do I tie a headscarf?" I wrote this book to answer that question, not only for chemotherapy patients, but for anyone who would like to tie a head wrap.

What inspired me?

I found myself looking around more and more at the way I saw headscarves tied, and not only at the women I saw in Day Oncology. I wondered at the beautiful way Mariam, my Somalian born friend, so gracefully tied hers. I saw people on the street using them as fashion items, and in winter their numbers multiplied as they warmed the heads of their wearers. There are millions of women (and men) around the world tying headwraps on their heads for different reasons. I discovered **Pinterest** and my horizons expanded! I have to admit I became infatuated with adding to my page **'*Headscarves, Head wraps and More*'** Everywhere they sold scarves I picked them up and handled them to evaluate their softness, elasticity, weaving, and general suitability for head wrapping. I assessed their pattern, colour, and price (and sometimes quickly put them down again!) Every time we went past an Op Shop (Australian for Charity Shop) I'd hear my husband groan, as I went rummaging through the donations for something suitable to exhibit in the book that was forming in my head. Whenever I saw someone wearing one I admired it, and took note of the way it matched clothing, or beautified the wearer.

Who I wrote it for

Whilst this book started with women undergoing chemo in mind, I realised that I wanted to reach others who love colour and pattern and playing with headscarves. I have not classed the styles as suitable for any one group. I would love this book to be read by **everyone** who wants to wrap – be it for health or culture, religion, modesty or fashion (and many other reasons I am sure).

Why I want people to read it

I hope that you pick this book up and admire all the styles, and pick at least a dozen ways *you* would like to tie a headwrap. I hope you pass by any ideas of head wraps being for other people, or ethnic groups, and see them as an extension of your personality. May you go out into your world wearing any of these styles with confidence and pizazz!

Finally - A great reason to buy this book

50% of the profits from books sold via **Cabrini Hospital**, *Brighton* and its sister hospitals in the area will go by private donation from me - the author, to help continue the giving of free wigs and headwear to those going through a vulnerable time.

Kaye Nutman
WRITER

Now... on to the styles!

3. Not your Granny's Knot

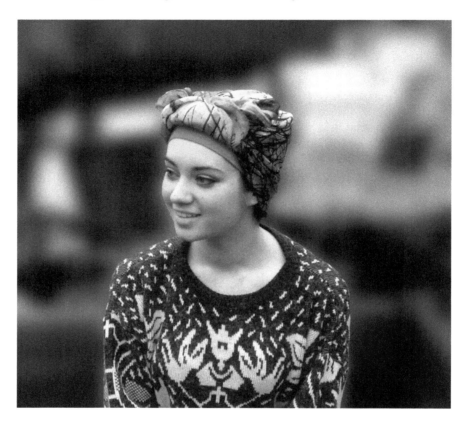

Not your Granny's Knot – Visual Instructions

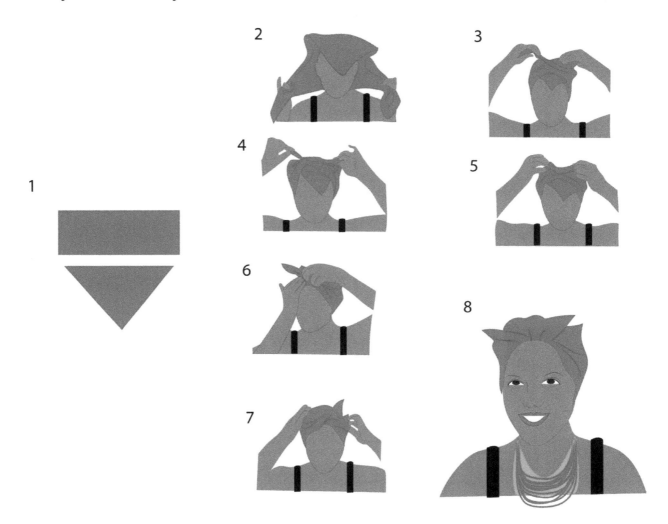

Not your Granny's Knot – Written Instructions

I tested out each set of Visual Instructions on my models, giving them no help – just asking them to choose a scarf and look at the pictures. The written instructions were available if they felt they needed to clarify something. The photograph here is Casey's 'take' on 'Not your Granny's Knot'.

Use a square scarf (the one in the photo is around 36"/90cm) and fold it corner to corner into a triangle. The one Casey used is one of my Op Shop finds. It is lovely and satiny, which allows it to drape into folds beautifully. She wore a hair band underneath, to help keep the silky scarf from slipping.

- Put the triangle over your head with the point centred over your nose and the long edge snug against the nape of your neck.

- Pull the two side corners forward and up to the top of your head. Cross over each other.

- Tie one knot. Then a second knot. Fluff the ends out into a bow.

- Pull the front point of the triangle gently, and fold it back over the centre of the bow, tucking it securely beneath the knot.

- Adjust the sides as needed.

- This looks great with some flattering lipstick and a cute necklace.

And you're done. Rock that look!

4. Simplicity Itself

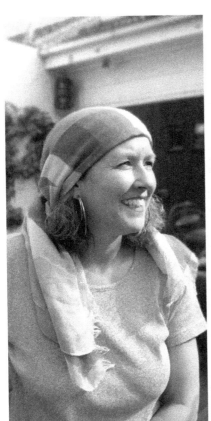 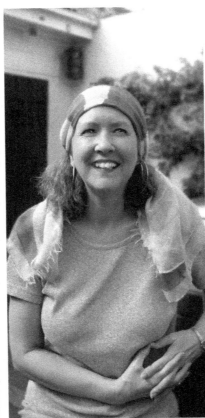 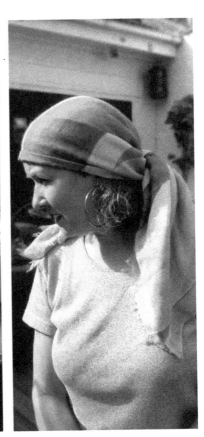

Simplicity Itself – Visual Instructions

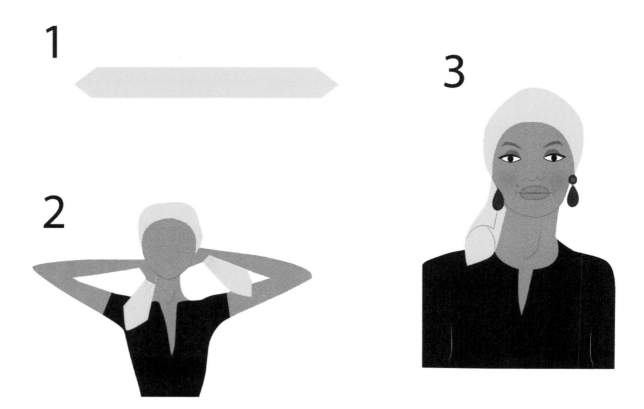

Simplicity Itself – Written Instructions

Don't be misled by Simplicity. This is the easiest headscarf tying idea, yet it can look fantastic.

Choose a material with slight stretch and it should stay put all day. You *can* use a velvet or textured headband underneath for added stability (with the nap running smooth down and rough texture upwards) or a lightweight cap.

The scarf in the photo of Anne was the first given to me by a good friend when I mentioned I was doing this book. It is long and wide, so I folded it in half length ways, then width ways. This gives great covering and an attractive casual layered look at the ends.

- Use a favourite long rectangular scarf or long piece of material.

- Place it over your head; centre at the forehead (each side should be of equal length), and make sure it comes down to the nape of your neck at the back.

- Tie once at the back, making sure any loose material is tucked behind the knot. Or you could also use an elastic hair tie to secure it.

- Adjust the forehead and ear height as desired. Pull the ends in front of your shoulders if long enough.

How easy is that?

Put on a dazzling pair of earrings to offset the Simplicity, or let the scarf take the limelight.

5. Go with the Flow

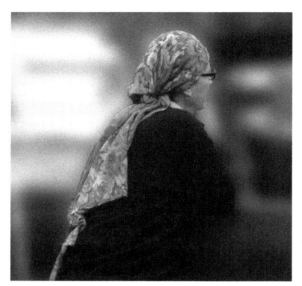 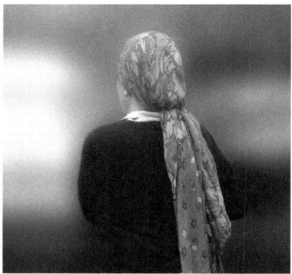

Go with the Flow – Visual Instructions

1

2

3

4

Go with the Flow – Written Instructions

This style uses a long rectangular scarf, and can be made with any fabric; it can be soft and flowy or crisp and neat in linen or cotton. My model Brigid chose a 100% polyester scarf which appears to float softly down her back.

If using a single colour you can really go to town on the accessories… headbands, flowers, brooches? Or make the scarf the star in a favourite multi-coloured pattern, like the one shown here.

No need to fold the edges under to fit the proportions of your head, though you *can* roll the front section under to give volume. The more that is left hanging, the 'flowier' it will appear.

- Swing the scarf behind your head, using both hands.

- Centre the front on your forehead.

- About 12" (30cm) from each side of your head, gather the scarf into a bunch (see Fig.2) and pull down and back to the nape of your neck.

- Cross the ends over the rest of the scarf and tie a single knot, then a second one. (Or you could use a hair tie wrapped firmly round the whole scarf when it is bunched together)

- Adjust at the forehead and around the ears; put on some long earrings.

Look over your shoulder and check in a long mirror to see how the scarf flows, and adjust as necessary. You can 'blouse' the top part out slightly, or go for a sleeker look.

6. Casual Elegance

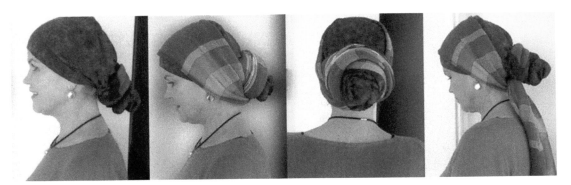

Casual Elegance – Visual Instructions

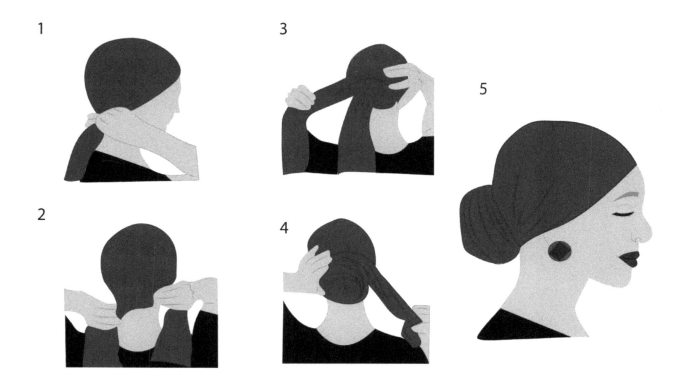

Casual Elegance – Written Instructions

This can be done with a rectangular scarf, or even two! My model, Michelle, chose two scarves that complemented the sweater she was wearing. How's this for ingenuity!

- Centre the scarf on your forehead and at the nape of your neck, with both sides of equal length. (Fold the scarf in, if it is too wide.)

- Cross the ends over at the nape of your neck, and tie. (You could use a hair tie for this step).

- Take one end of the scarf in one hand, and start wrapping it round and round *tightly* going underneath the other hanging end. Use your second hand to help keep the tension up, until it forms a tight bun. Tuck the end in.

- Now take the hanging end and twist it round the first bun you made. Tuck that in too. If you want more security and your scarf isn't too precious – like silk, you can use a bobby pin where the bun meets the scarf underneath, or you can use a hair tie near the base.

Now it's time for the 'lippy', makeup and jewellery.

See what effect a second scarf can have on the wrap:

Fold one, in a complementary colour, into a band, and then wrap it around your head. Cross over underneath, then round the bun. Tuck in and tidy. Or you can leave it dangling down your back, like Michelle did in the last photo, for a more casual look.

7. Simply Does It

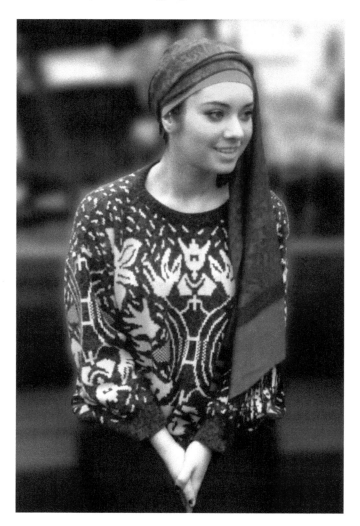

Simply Does It – Visual Instructions

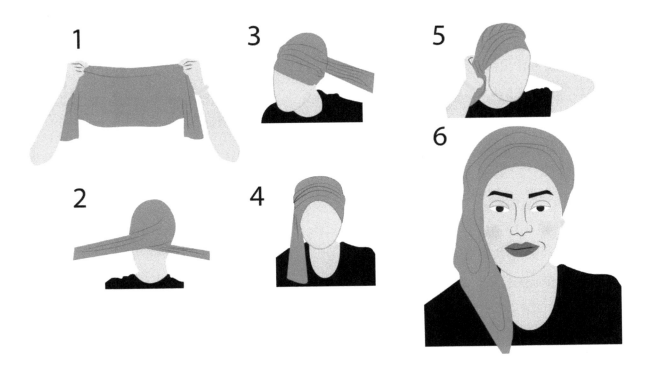

Simply Does It – Written Instructions

For this wrap, Casey chose a fabulous pinky purple Tichel which I bought last year from the website www.wrapunzel.com . She likes to wear a head band underneath, and I think she looks oh so chic in it. In fact, it reminds me *a bit* of 'Girl with a Pearl Earring' – though it's not blue and gold!

- Take a long rectangular scarf and fold it over lengthways for the correct fit between the nape of the neck and the middle of the forehead.

- Centre the scarf on your head. Flick the ends over each shoulder, to the back. Take hold of each side. Pass one side over the other, and tighten the scarf to comfortably hug the head.

- Pull one end of the scarf over the head. You may give one or more gentle twist as you go. Pull the other end of the scarf to the front of your shoulder.

- Tie the two ends together at the side, above your ear. Adjust the edges of the scarf over your ears.

- You could push the shorter end of the scarf under at the back of your head.

- Tease the other end so that it flattens out around the knot, pull it in front of your shoulder. Admire yourself in the mirror! Don't you love it?

8. Braided Wonder

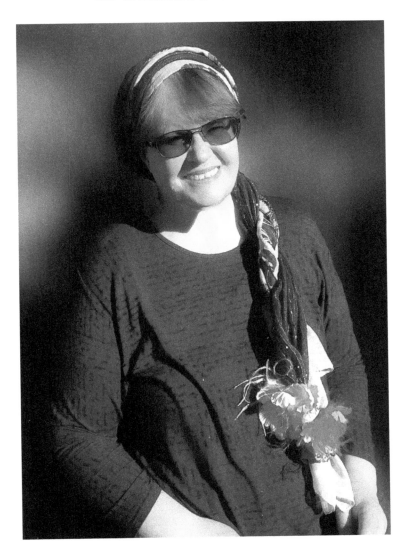

Braided Wonder – Visual Instructions

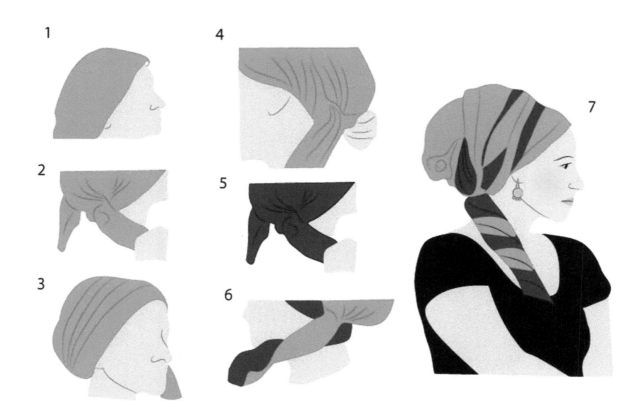

Braided Wonder – Written Instructions

Not as difficult as it looks! Stun your friends with this amazing look and have them all asking for a demonstration! This style uses two of your longest scarves of about the same thickness. Have a hair tie handy at the end. (Put it round your wrist, ready to slide it off, straight on to the end of the 'braid'.) You could use a volumiser underneath for more height at the back.

- Place scarf 1 on your head. Two thirds should fall to one side, 1/3 to the other.

- Tie it in a simple knot at the back.

- Grip the knot and pull gently to the side. The scarf should follow it round.

- Pull gently on each length to tighten any folds and flatten the knot.

- Fold scarf 2 in half. Repeat the first four instructions, leaving some of scarf 1 exposed at the front.

- Wrap both lengths of scarf 1 over your head 2cm or so behind scarf 2. Repeat with the other scarf. Now pull the ends gently back to the side and put each colour together.

- If the scarves are really long, you can go round again... then

- Braid the scarves, by wrapping over each other. (It is helpful to be looking in the mirror as you do this, so you can smooth it out as you go along) If the shorter lengths run out, push them under the longer lengths and keep going. Pop a hair tie – plain or fancy – on the end.

Pat used two flower clips to add pizzazz. There is a certain 'Bo-Ho' look to this style.

9. Easy Peasy Wrap n Roll

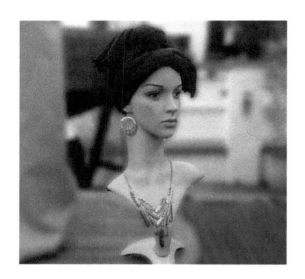 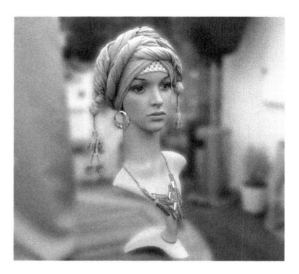

Visual Instructions – Easy Peasy Wrap n Roll

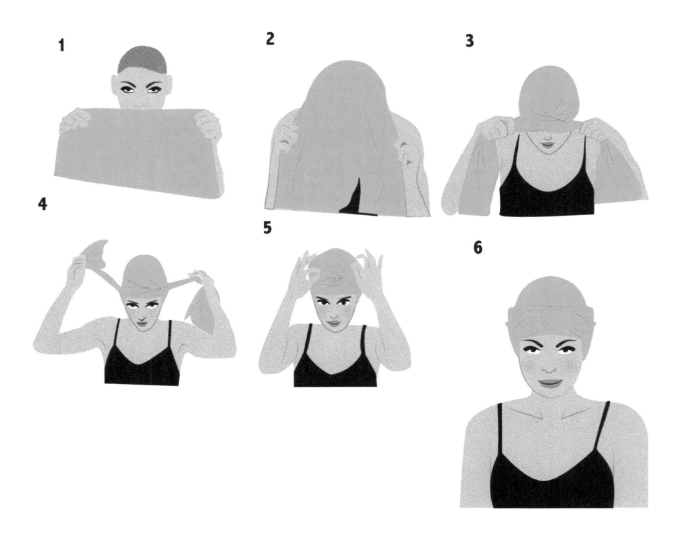

Written Instructions – Easy Peasy Wrap n Roll

You can use a Rectangular scarf with a little stretch. Jersey, Rayon or Cotton would be a good choice. If you want to wear a scarf cap underneath, this could be in a contrasting colour and peek out a little or be totally hidden. You can use tassels or bobbles for a Bo Ho look.

- Hold the scarf in front of you and find the centre of the long edge. You can fold part of the scarf back on itself to create the correct width between your forehead and the nape of your neck.

- Lean your head forward and place the folded edge of the scarf around the nape of your neck and have the edges hanging in front of your body.

- Slide your hands a little further down the scarf on each side, grasp the material and pinch each side into one piece. Criss-Cross the pieces firmly over your forehead, catching the front of the scarf underneath.

- Twist each strand as you take it round to the back of your head, (wrap n roll) cross them over each other and continue round to the front.

- Tie the two ends together above the centre of your forehead - into a double knot, or a bow. Tuck in any loose edges or ends, unless you want them as part of a casual design (Bo-Ho look!).

- Check that the front edge of the scarf is at the most attractive forehead height for you and covers your ears (leaving the earlobes on display), and that the twists and knot created look as neat or as casual as you desire.

Wow! That's a great look.

10. Creative Crossover

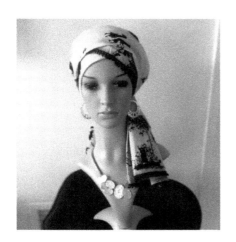 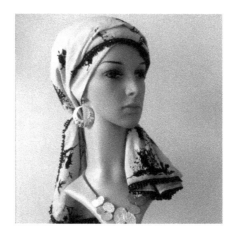

Creative Crossover – Visual Instructions.

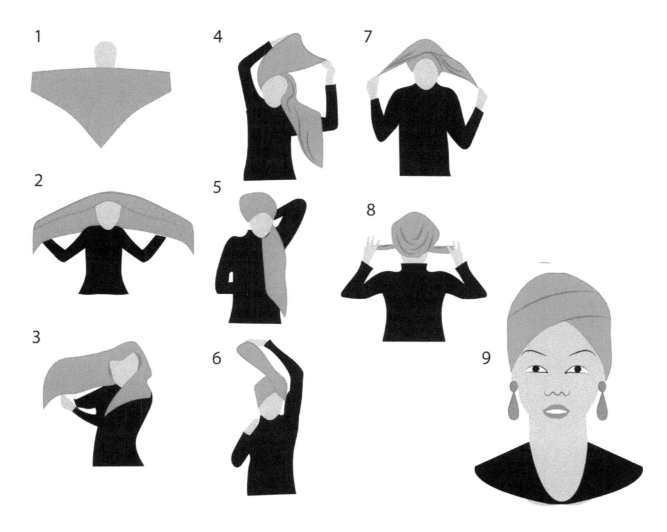

Creative Crossover – Written Instructions

A very versatile wrap. It can be styled with a large square scarf (folded into a triangle), or a rectangular one. My illustrations show a triangle, but I've dressed Eddie in a rectangular one. This can be worn with the ends tucked in or left hanging out, to protect the back of the neck. It makes up well in many different materials, and looks great with a scarf edged in a contrasting colour to show the symmetry of the style.

- Fold your square, corner to corner diagonally, into a triangle.

- Centre the triangle on your head, with the short point at the back.

- Pull each long end forward in front of your shoulders.

- Pull one side diagonally up, over and to the back of your head.

- Allow it to hang down the back

- Pull the second side diagonally up, over your forehead. This results in a nice cross over at the front. It should be directly in line with your nose.

- Take each end in your hands and cross over at the nape of your neck, over the short pointed end. (If using a rectangular scarf you can probably do this once more, and then tie.)

- Tuck the ends firmly under at the back; this looks neat. Or just tuck in the pointed end, to leave a more casual neck covering, as in the photo.

You can now choose to put on some earrings, or keep it simple.

Tip: If you are used to a side parting, then you can do the front crossover above an eyebrow.

11.Round n r Round

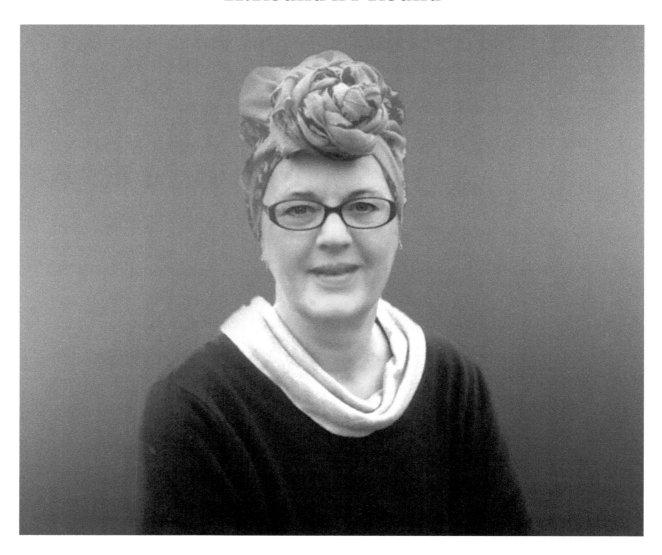

Round n r Round – Visual Instructions

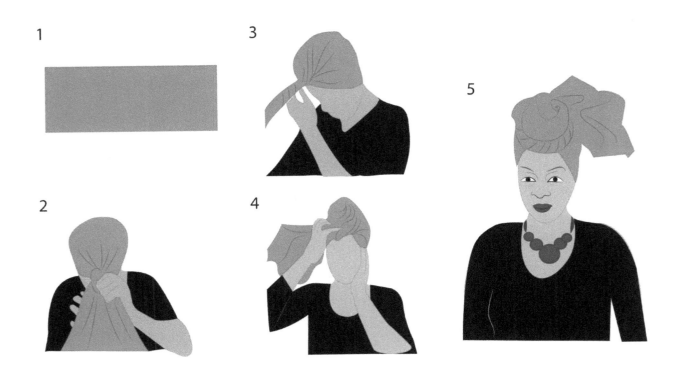

Round n r Round – Written Instructions

Use one of your long rectangular scarves in a lightweight or mid weight material; the heavier the material the larger the bun, in general.

- Take your long scarf and turn back one edge so that it will fit neatly over the head, from forehead to the nape of the neck.

- Place it on the centre of your head with both sides of even length. Pull each side to the front, so the back is snug at the nape of your neck, and tie once on your forehead, tucking in any loose bits behind the knot.

- Twist the two ends together TIGHTLY, round and round, almost to the end.

- Now, twist the 'rope' you have made round and round in a tight circular motion, using your free hand to stabilise the bun as it is made.

- Tuck the end underneath the bun –it can be pushed in fully for a neat look (as in the photo of Brigid) or you can push the rope underneath the bun further back along its length, and allow the end to fluff out in an attractive casual manner.

Now, add make-up and accessories, and walk out the door feeling confident, fashionable and like a million dollars!.

Like to see an example on video? Have a look on YouTube

Ref: Eva's Head-wraps #5   http://tinyurl.com/zasrc3b

You can look along the right hand side of the screen for similar videos.

12.   Buffed Up Bun

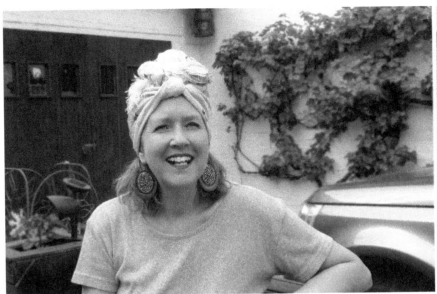 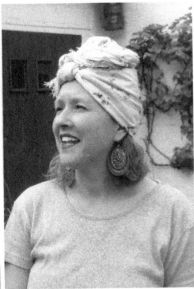

Buffed Up Bun – Visual Instructions

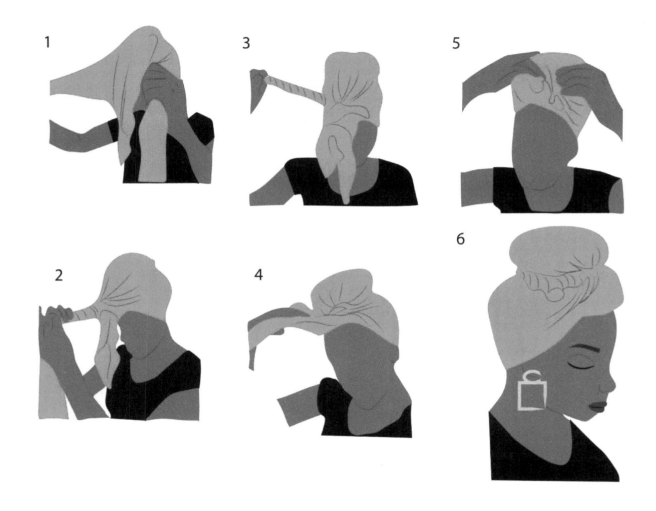

Buffed Up Bun – Written Instructions

With long hair - tie it into a bun on *top* of your head. If you have no hair or have short hair – try this... Take a scarf and roll it loosely into a ball about the size of a bun. Place it on the crown of your head. Have a second scarf ready – a square folded into a triangle.

- Centre the long edge of the scarf at the nape of your neck, with the middle point passing over the bun and falling onto your face. Pull the two long corner edges to the front.

- Cross these over firmly at the front; keep the short point of the scarf underneath. Adjust the 'bun' to make sure it sits neatly on the crown of your head. Twist the two long pieces round each other tightly, to form one long rope.

- Wrap the rope all the way around the bun; tuck the end in securely.

- Take the point covering your face and twist it round loosely.

- Secure the front point in the rope surrounding the bun. Adjust the front to sit neatly.

- Put on your make-up and a great pair of earrings.

So elegant! If you have long hair a few stray wisps will soften the look for casual styling.

You could also add volume using a false bun bought from a hair care shop, as shown here by Pat.

Tip: Other ideas for adding volume are given in a Section 2.

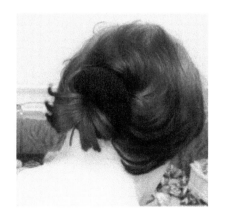

13.   Put it All Behind You

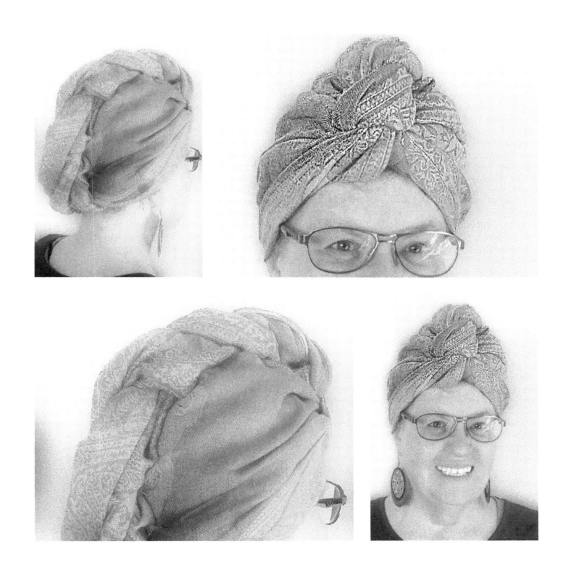

Put it all Behind You – Visual Instructions

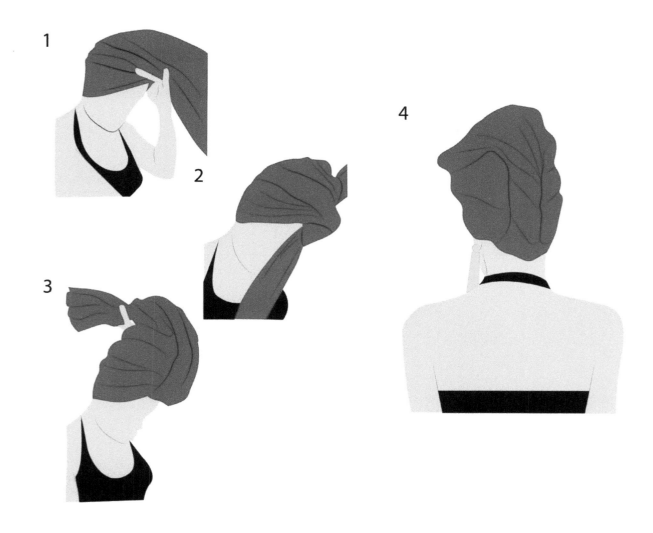

Put it All Behind You – Written Instructions

This style is *great* for giving height. It really suits a round face, elongating the portrait and profile, but equally suits any shape. It makes up beautifully in a thicker material, a pashmina, or any long rectangular shape.

- Centre the scarf at the back of the head, curving round the nape of your neck. Push all the material to the front and grip at the centre of your forehead.

- You *can* tie knot to keep the scarf comfortably secure, or hold it tightly before the next step. Adjust it over the ears and at your hairline.

- Twist gently.as you pull the material from front to back along the centre line of your head. Check in the mirror to see if it is lined up with your nose.

- Give a few extra twists from the crown of your skull to the nape of the neck and tuck in securely.

This is such a simple, yet flattering style. Decide on the shape of earrings you will wear to complement the look; swipe on some lipstick and a little eyeliner and you're good to go!

Sophisticated when dressing up for evening or casual for daytime, depending on the scarf you choose.

14.   Terrific Triangle

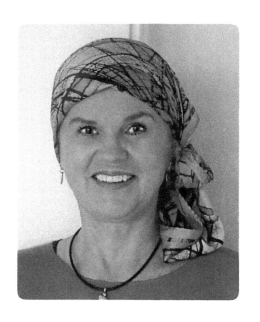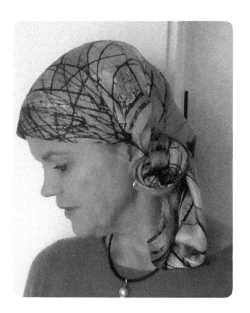

Terrific Triangle – Visual Instructions

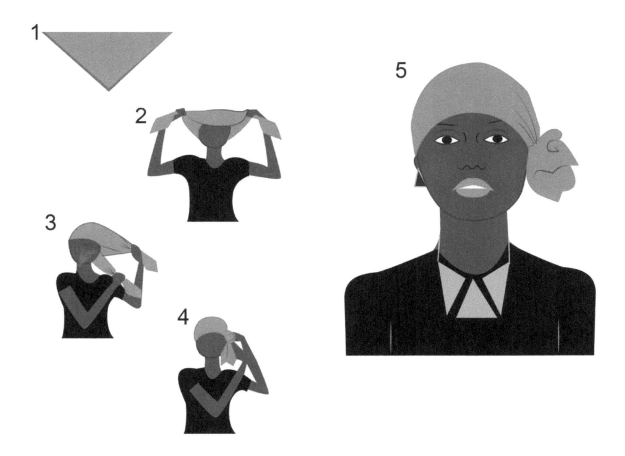

Terrific Triangle – Written Instructions

Another triangle based style. Use a small or medium square scarf in a flowing fabric for a flattering effect, or a crisper material for volume at the side. If the scarf is satiny or silk then you may want to put a velvet headband underneath (rough going upwards, smooth side down) to give the material more grip.

- Fold your square into a triangle.

- Grab the corners on the longest edge and centre the scarf over your head, at the desired height on your forehead. The shorter pointed edge is behind you.

- Push one end behind your shoulder, then reach round and grab it, so that both ends are on one side. Make sure you go over the top of the short point.

- Use a gentle pulling motion to make the two ends an equal length.

- Tie once at the side of your head, just behind your ear. Adjust the positioning of the scarf over the other ear, at the nape of your neck and on your forehead.

- Tie again, into a bow. The loops and ends will cascade gently down if a soft material is used, or will stand up crisply with a firmer material (fiddle and adjust to your liking).

Match the colour to your outfit, or go bold and funky. The choice is yours! Look in a mirror and add earrings and lipstick. How flattering is this?

15.Fun with Knots

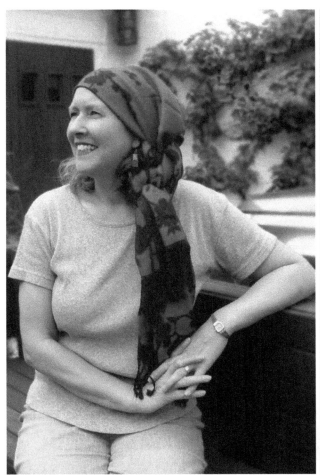
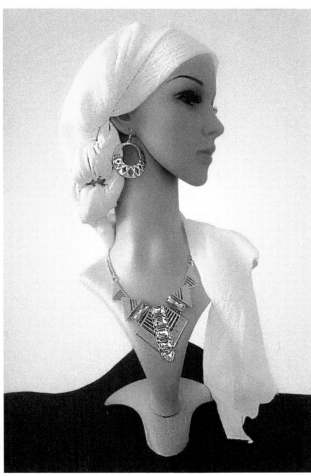

Fun with Knots – Visual Instructions

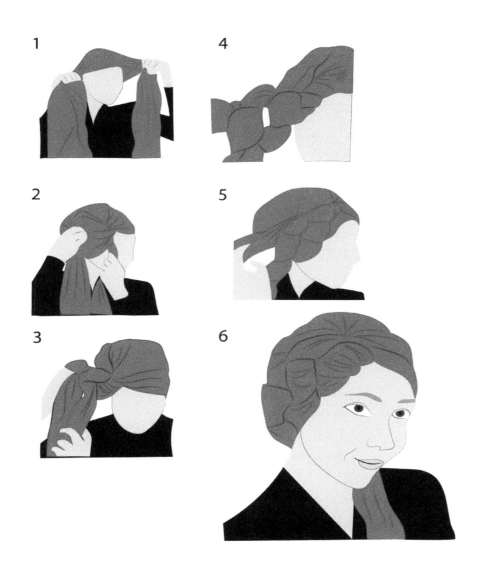

Fun with Knots – Written Instructions

Lightweight, medium weight or heavyweight material? This can make the difference between an elegant, casual or fun look - and this wrap looks great with them all. There is also a secret in the tying. This head wrap can take you from day to evening in just a few knots.

- Start by centring a long rectangular scarf on your head, covering from the nape of the neck to the forehead. Both sides should be equal in length. Hold firmly in each hand, and a little way from the ears.

- Gently slide the scarf around your head until your hands meet on one side, above the eyebrow. Tie a firm knot. Check that the back covers the nape of the neck, and the front is at a pleasing height, and covers the ears.

- Smooth the ends for a tidy look, or leave crinkled for a more casual, thicker knotted look. Hold the two ends out to the side and tie a second knot.

- Put in a third knot and assess if there is room for more. Tie another knot and take the 'rope' you have made round to the back of your head.

- Keep knotting until the rope reaches the centre of your neck at the back. You can tuck the ends under if you have used a short scarf, or...

- If there is still room, add knots until the 'rope' reaches over the opposite shoulder. Secure the ends together with a hair tie, so the knots stay in shape.

Another version of this is to tie the first knot behind the ear, and treat it like a plait (braid), casually thrown over the opposite shoulder.

16. Side Bun Sensation

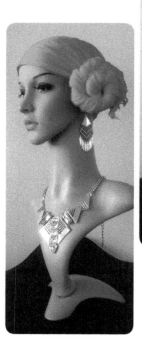
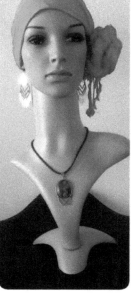
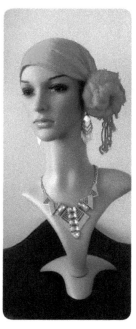

Side Bun Sensation – Visual Instructions

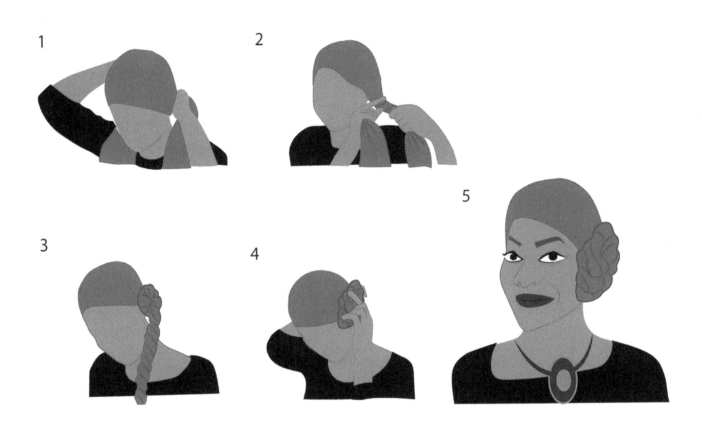

Side Bun Sensation – Written Instructions

Choosing a plain rectangular scarf for this style will show off the clever twisting action, though patterned scarves look beautiful too.

(A bunch of buns)

- Place the scarf centrally on your head; adjust the front to the height on your forehead which is most flattering to you. Gather both pieces together at the back.

- Pull both pieces to one side and over the shoulder to the front. Adjust so that they are of equal length. Twist each piece as you go, and cross it over the other piece; this twisting action results in a neat but showy bun.

- Once the rope is completed take it above the ear and start to wrap it round into a tight circle.

- Continue the wrapping process until you reach the end of the rope. Tuck in tightly.

Make those eyes pop when you apply your make-up, and add accessories such as glamourous earrings and necklace for an evening look. Fabulous!

Take a look at this video: Sisi Yemmie - (start at 0.33seconds to skip the promo part) https://youtu.be/Uo3wcJdf4yc

17. Effortless Beauty

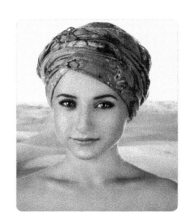
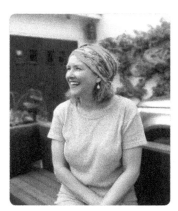
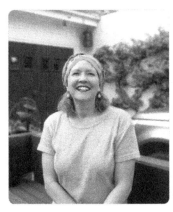
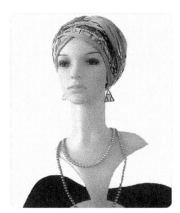

Effortless Beauty – Visual Instructions

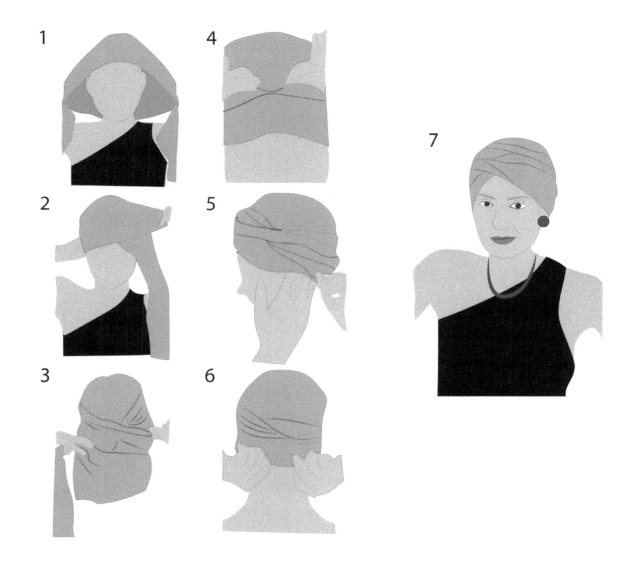

Effortless Beauty – Written Instructions

Lovely Anne, came to the rescue here with my photography. This is a graceful style that I often show to clients in my volunteer capacity in Day Oncology. It could be called The 10 Second Wrap. There are several variations that only take a few seconds longer. Fold the scarf before you begin so that it will fit snugly between your forehead and the nape of your neck. If there is a border to the scarf make sure it shows.

- Centre the scarf on your head so that it is equal on both sides. Hold out each side like you have your hair in bunches.
- Pull one side round and diagonally across your forehead, let the other end dangle. Smooth the pleating so that it sits neatly on your head.
- Pull the other side up and diagonally across your forehead. Adjust so that the cross over is in line with your nose. (If you like your hair with a side parting, you could align the cross over with your right or left eye, as in the 'desert sands' picture.) Cross the ends over at the base of your neck.
- Pull the ends round to the front, keeping any folds in the material smooth and flat. Cross over again if there is enough length.
- Tuck the ends into the edges of the first crossover that you made. Adjust the outer edges of the scarf to an attractive level, leaving room to see any earrings you may wear.
- If the scarf is long you may need to wrap it round to the back, and tuck in underneath at the nape of the neck. Run your hands around all edges of the scarf for a neat, classic look.

How about picking a colour from the scarf and matching it to lips, or earrings and necklace? Play around until you get the look you desire.

18. Happily Harmonious

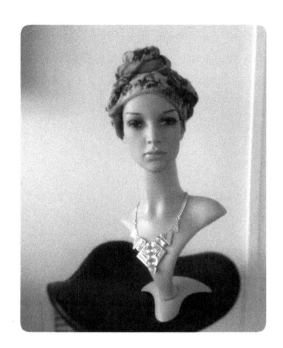 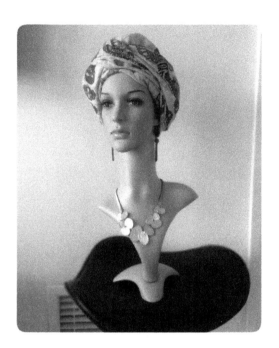

Add volume to your style with this double wrap technique

Happily Harmonious – Visual Instructions

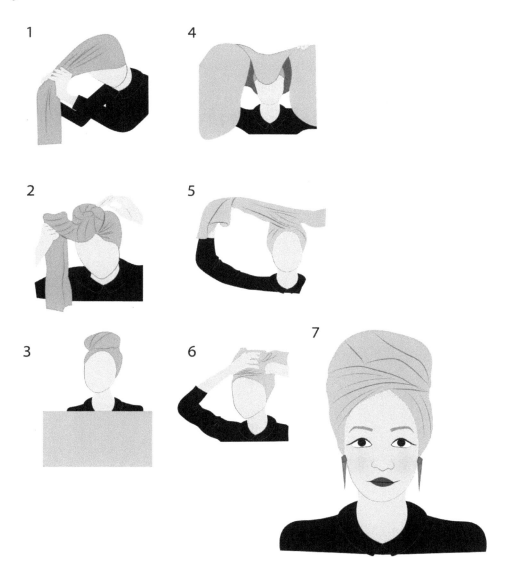

Happily Harmonious – Written Instructions

This wrap uses two scarves to achieve height. It builds on Wraps 9 and 14 to create an illusion of copious amounts of hair hidden underneath. If you *do* have long hair, a few strands peeking out around the edges can add softness to the look.

You can use a mid-weight scarf underneath and a lighter weight on top, or have fun and experiment with different weights of material. Even though the under scarf won't be seen, it feels nice to have toning colours.

- Take a long scarf and turn back one edge so that it will fit neatly over your head, from forehead to the nape of the neck. Place it on the centre of the head with both sides of even length. Pull each side to the front at forehead height.

- Twist the two ends together tightly, round and round, almost to the end.

- Now, wrap the 'rope' you have made round and round in a circular motion, using the free hand to stabilize the bun as it is made. Tuck the end under the bun.

- Take your second scarf and centre it over your head. Make sure it covers the nape of your neck, the bun and sits on your forehead at the desired height.

- Do a simple crossover of the two ends, at the front, keeping it firm.

- Wrap it round to the back, cross over again and bring to back to the front. Tuck the ends in neatly.

- Adjust the edges. Apply lipstick and earrings.

There you have it; a harmonious wrap to be proud of!

19. Brilliant Braid

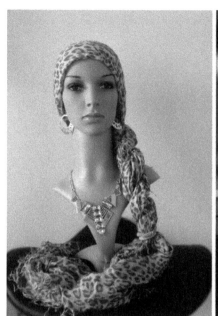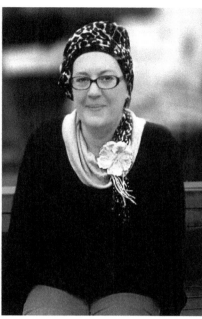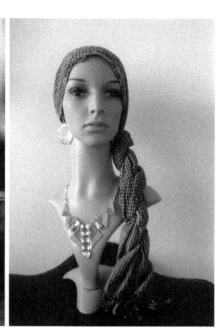

Brilliant Braid – Visual Instructions

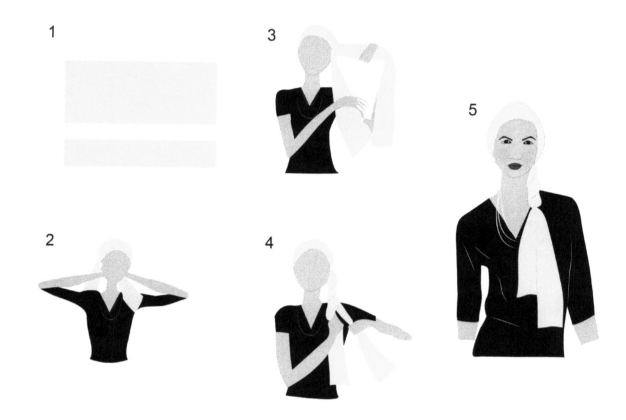

1

2

3

4

5

Brilliant Braid – Written Instructions

If you like, you can use a cotton cap underneath this scarf; a coloured swimming cap (in material, not rubber) could be used also. This works best with a scarf with a little bit of stretch – such as viscose. Slip a hair tie over one wrist in readiness.

- Take a long rectangular scarf and fold it in half, or to the desired width. Make sure it will cover the back of your head fully.

- With the folded edge of the scarf centred at the front, place the scarf over your head. Push the ends behind you and tie firmly. Adjust the edges comfortably over the ears.

- Gently pull both long ends of the scarf to the desired side, and hold one in each hand.

- Twist the edges over each other (not together – they would simply unwind).

- Keep going until you reach the desired length or until the scarf runs out. Slip the hair tie from your wrist onto the scarf to secure the ends. This leaves a lovely braided effect.

- Decorate with a flower or ribbon in a contrasting colour if you desire.

This can look school girl cute or grown-up sophisticated depending on what you add to the style. Certainly a dash of lipstick and swipe of eyeliner will enhance the look, as would earrings, a necklace or both.

20. CanTeen Casey

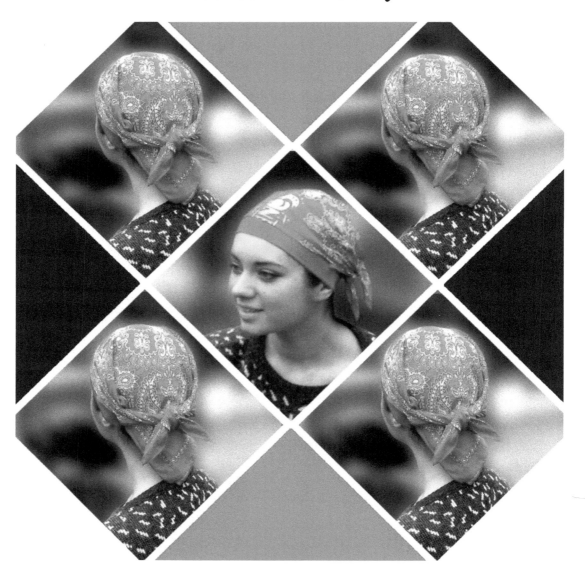

CanTeen Casey – Visual Instructions

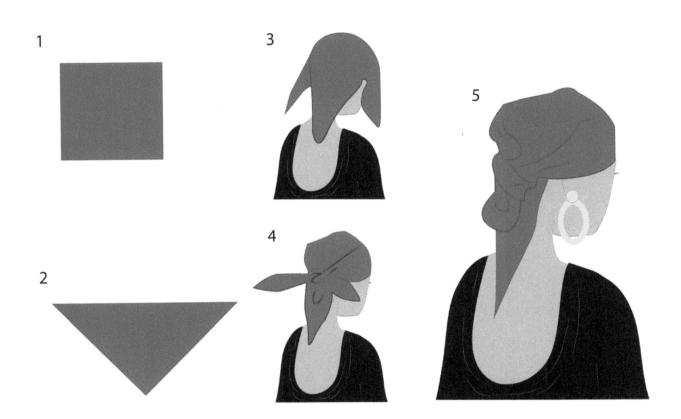

CanTeen Casey – Written Instructions

Here in Australia we have something called 'National Bandana Day'. In the weeks leading up to it, some supermarkets have displays of coloured bandanas, like the one that Casey wears in the photo. Many schools encourage the students to wear one on the day, so this is a great awareness raiser for Children's Cancers, and a fundraiser for CanTeen, a registered charity in Australia. I'm sure there is something similar in many countries.

Of course, bandanas are also trendy items to wear all year round! This style works as well with silky materials, as with cotton; a hair band or under cap can extend the width and give the wearer more coverage.

- Take a small square scarf.

- Fold it into a triangle.

- Place the triangle over the head, centred at the forehead, middle point down the back.

- Tie a knot over the middle point at the nape of the neck.

- If there is enough material, tie a bow - if not, then another knot. Pull gently above the knot to puff the scarf out a little, and check how the front looks.

Now, accessorise with a great pair of earrings – hoops can look fantastically pirate-y!

You're all set.

21.   Pump up the Volume

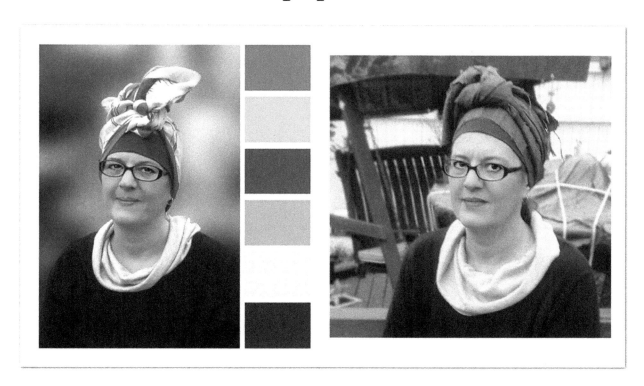

Pump up the Volume – Visual Instructions

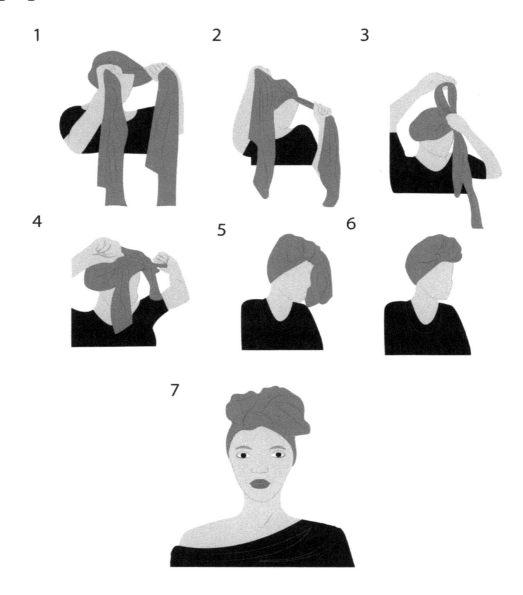

Pump up the Volume – Written Instructions

- Using a long rectangular scarf place it over your head. The side lengths should be equal. The front should be centred on the forehead. Gripping both side lengths, just above your shoulders, pull to the front. The back should cradle the base of your skull.

- Cross the side lengths over in front of your forehead. Take the length underneath and pull it up and through the gap to create a knot. Pull the ends firmly.

- Make the first loop of a bow by pulling the centre of the right side length upwards and grip the base of the loop with that hand.

- Pull the left side of the scarf around the loop and your hand in a circle. Use the fingertips of the right hand to pull the scarf through the gap to make a second loop. (Hold the loop already made, in your left hand so that you can tug the second loop through.)

- Fan out both loops gently, so that they are equal.

- Pull any excess scarf length loosely over the centre of the bow and tuck in securely.

You nailed it!

22. Trouble Free Triangle

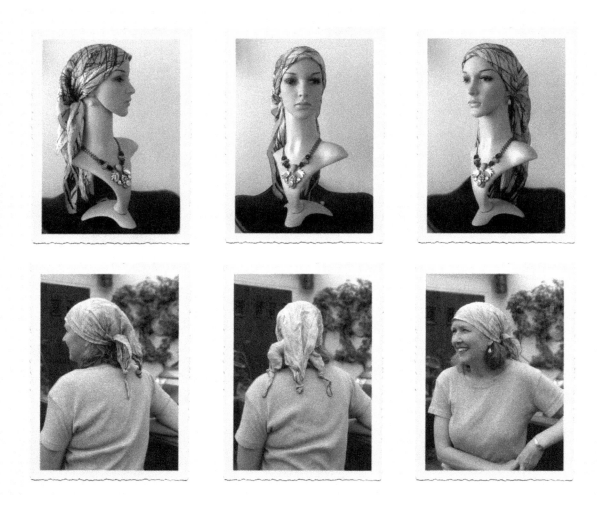

Trouble Free Triangle – Visual Instructions

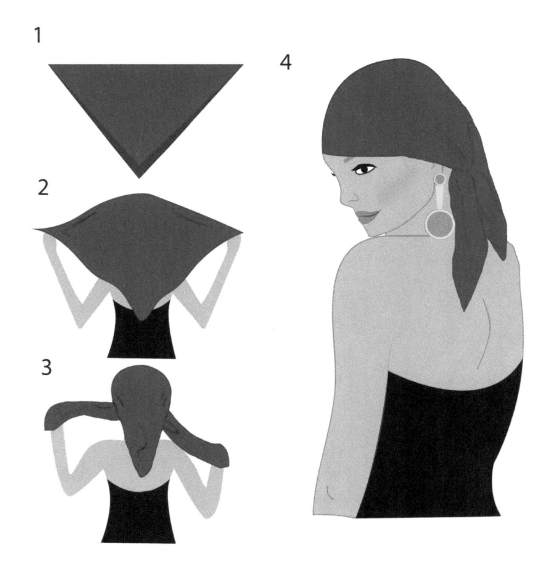

1

2

3

4

Trouble Free Triangle – Written Instructions

Crisp cotton, stretch jersey or silky satin with a velvet headband underneath - all work fabulously. Plain, patterned, or edged material; this really is a versatile style. Wear it with panache!

- Fold a small or medium size square scarf in half diagonally, to form a triangle. Try to match up each corner.

- Turn back a few cm/inches along the length of the longest edge. This gives the front a bit of volume.

- Hold the two points at either end and put the centre on your forehead, with the shorter point hanging down at the back.

- Flip the short point over to the front of your head to keep it out of the way.

- Tie the two long ends together in a firm knot at the back of your neck.

- Flip the middle point back, to cover the knot you just made.

- Arrange the scarf at the desired height above your eyes and over your ears. All three points of the scarf should hang comfortably down at the back.

Add simple jewellery to show off this simple style. If you have used a flowing material, try tying a knot in each of the three ends, like Anne has, for a funky casual look.

23. Fanciful Fun

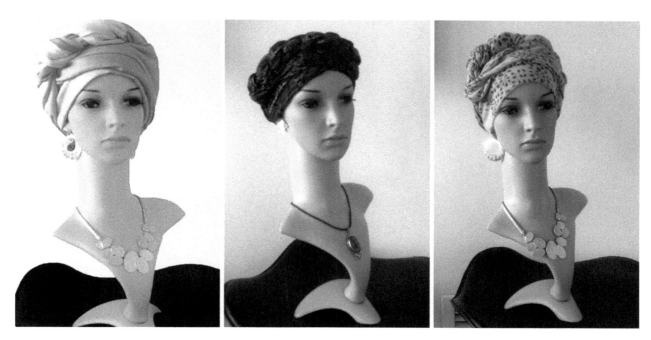

Fanciful Fun – Visual Instructions

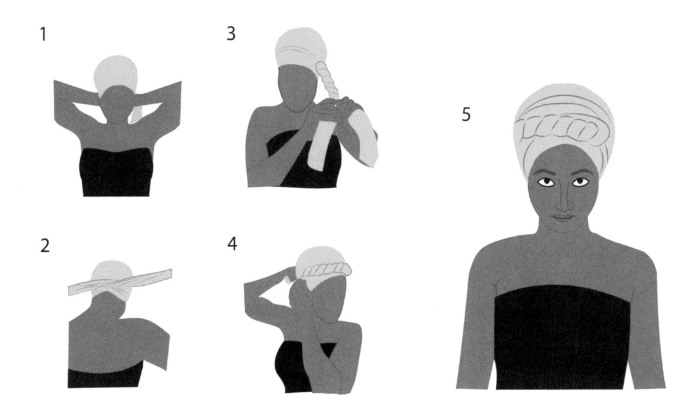

Fanciful Fun – Written Instructions

I soooo fell in love with this style! I dressed up Eddie, my mannequin, in several different scarf weights and patterns. This is a sure fire winner, and bound to get people asking you how you did it.

Use a long rectangular scarf and turn in the edge to get the right width to cover from forehead to the nape of your neck.

- Start with the scarf over your head, from forehead to the nape of your neck. Each side should be of equal length at this point.

- Cross over smoothly at the back then pull both ends round to the forehead.

- Adjust the ends to meet just above the temple on one side, and cross one over the other. Pull the rope in front of you so you can see what you are doing. Wrap the ends around each other to make a neat, tight, rope.

- Pull the rope upwards and across the forehead, and tuck the ends into the gap between two layers at the opposite side.

- Adjust the scarf over the ears and check that the rope end is firmly tucked in. Smile at yourself in the mirror, put on some make-up, and go out and Wow your friends.

Ref: Eva's Head-wraps #6   https://www.youtube.com/watch?v=SAxY_86CE3I

24. Safe n Secure

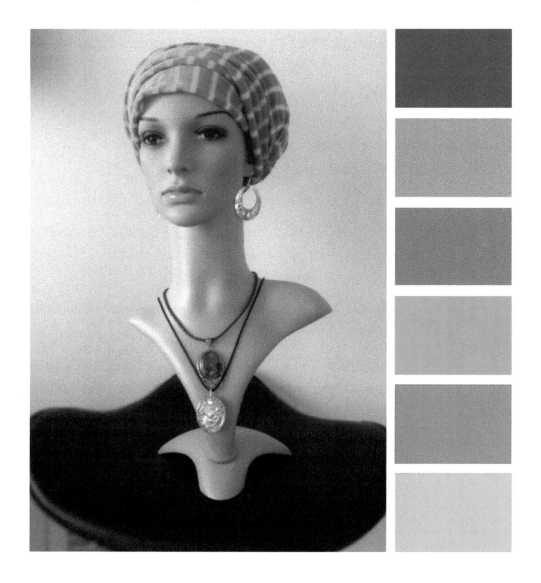

Safe n Secure – Visual Instructions

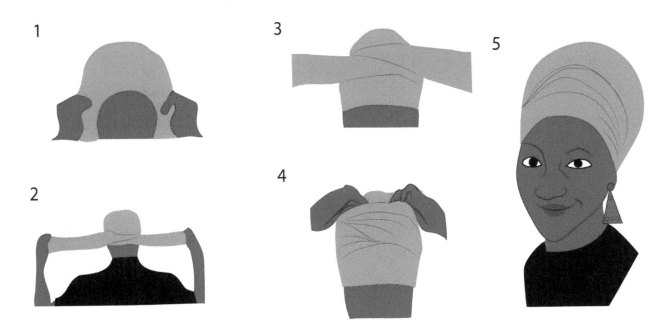

Safe n Secure – Written Instructions

Use a long rectangular scarf for this style. Fold it over lengthways, so that is a long narrow rectangle which fits neatly between your forehead and the nape of your neck. For the photo we used a stretch jersey scarf.

- Centre the wrap on your head with the tails of the scarf behind your shoulders.

- Cross the ends over firmly at the back, at the nape of your neck, pulling the ends out to the sides.

- Pull firmly round to the front, catching the back of the scarf underneath, and cross over 1"/2-3cm above the edge of the scarf on your forehead.

- If the scarf is long enough, go round to the back, cross over tightly again and tuck in the ends at the front. If it is not long enough, tuck them in at the back.

- Time to get out the eye liner and lipstick, and a striking pair of earrings.

If you want to add more glamour, look out for a jewelled brooch which matches the tone of your scarf and earrings, and place it at the side or in the centre of the scarf at the front.

25. Ticheled Pink (or Damson and Green)

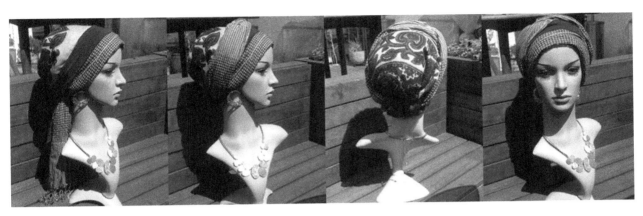

Tichel (pronounced *tick*-el – or close!). I used a Volumiser to give extra padding beneath this (pseudo) Tichel, since 'Eddie' has no hair. Check out Section 2 to see how wonderful they really look.

Ticheled Pink – Visual Instructions

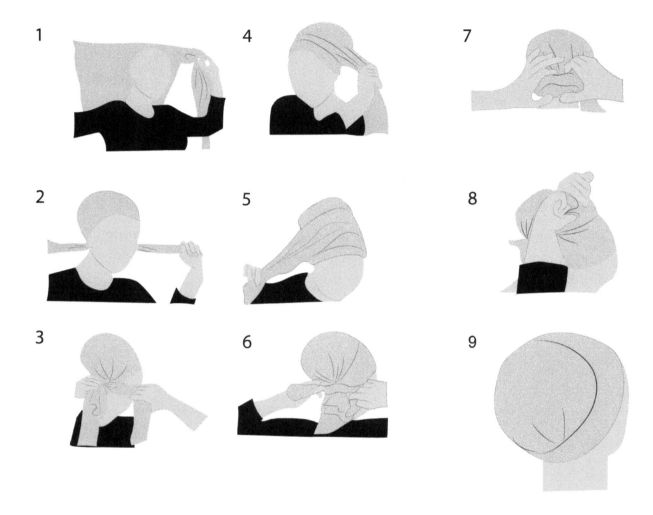

Ticheled Pink – Written Instructions

I got this idea when I saw an Apron Tichel on Pinterest; Since I didn't have one of these scarves myself, I adapted the idea. *This style looks great with a Volumiser.

I used a large square scarf folded into quarters. Then I took a long thin rectangular scarf and folded it in half to make it thinner - then lay that on top to make the apron shape (think waisted apron, not bib type).

- Place the scarves over your head; centre at the forehead.

- Push the 'apron strings' behind your shoulders and cross over loosely at the nape of your neck – *on top* of the first scarf. Smooth the back of the scarf to neaten the appearance, pull the 'apron strings' tight, and knot.

- Pull one end of the narrower scarf (apron strings) across the front of the head, smoothing as you go.

- Pull the other end of the narrower scarf neatly round and over in the opposite direction. If the scarf is particularly long, then go round again.

- Push the two narrow ends in securely at the nape of the neck. Gently tug down, then fold up any of the remaining material from the square scarf and tuck in over the top of the knot you made.

This is designed to be a neat, modest style; now you can add a stretchy circular hair-band to give an accent colour, if you wish. Add make-up and accessories and you're good to go!

Check out the Section 2 to see how a Tichel is worn by Rivka Malka. Volumisers are shown there too.

26. Zigger-Zag Criss-Cross

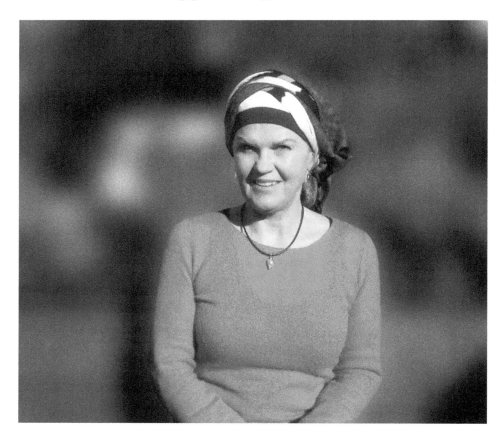

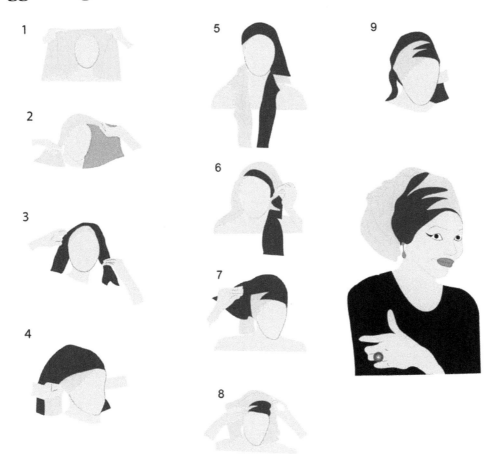

Zigger-Zag Criss-Cross– Visual Instructions

Zigger-Zag Criss-Cross – Written Instructions

This appears to have a lot of steps, but don't worry – you can do it! If you like precision, you'll love this. You will need two very long rectangular scarves. This looks fantastic with different coloured plain scarves, or one plain, one patterned – experiment with what you have. Michelle's first attempt at this really nailed it!

- Make sure the first scarf is centred on your head, and the ends are of equal length.
- Angle one side at the front so it sits with the scarf covering your ear, the other end goes behind the ear on the opposite side. Tie together at the nape of your neck.
- Take the second scarf and place it at an angle over the first - in the opposite direction. The crossover should be level with your nose.
- Tie at the back, *underneath* the first scarf and its tails.
- Push one end of each scarf to the front of your shoulder.
- Take the end of scarf 1 that is hanging at the back, and bring it over your head, at an angle – match it up with the first criss-cross. Keep it flat and tidy. Let the end hang to the back.
- Take the second scarf end from the back; cross over the head at an angle, matching the intersection below. Let this end hang down at the back too.
- Take scarf 1 (the end hanging in front of your shoulder) and pull it up and over to the other side, crossing over diagonally in line with the nose. You should cross over the end from scarf two but leave it hanging out at the back.
- Take scarf 2 (the end in front of your shoulder) and repeat the last step. You now have four ends hanging out at the back, but a pretty neat looking front.
- Criss-cross the ends at the back and tuck them in. Look in two mirrors (one in front, one behind). You will find a very attractive back view. You could leave two hanging ends out. Done! Easier than you thought – eh?

27. SECTION TWO

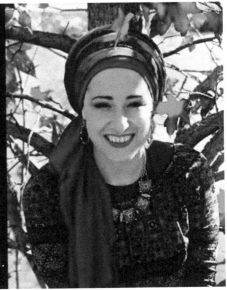

We live in such an important time, and women
hold the key to change
and redemption.
Can you feel what I mean?
There's a clippity-clop of footsteps, an urgency,
a desire to achieve
our potential
and to live
at our highest capacity both personally and
professionally.

Rivka Malka Perlman
Transformative Life Coach and co-founder of Wrapunzel.

I was going to fill a few pages with inspiring quotes as well as information – but, sadly, I lack the space! So, this is a favourite quote of mine from one of the founders of the website 'Wrapunzel'. The website is now run by co-founder Andrea Grinberg. Check out http://www.wrapunzel.com/ for more great examples of how a Tichel can look *fabulous* for *everyone!* Check along the top bar, and on the side bar, for access to the blog. (I love 'Lady Wrap Stars') Find video tutorials, (see the *Zig-Zag Criss-Cross* tutorial – third one in, on the Tutorials page) http://www.wrapunzel.com/tutorials/ and all kinds of other interesting items.

Other good places to look for scarf ideas are on Etsy, eBay and by Googling Headscarf websites for your country.

Volumisers

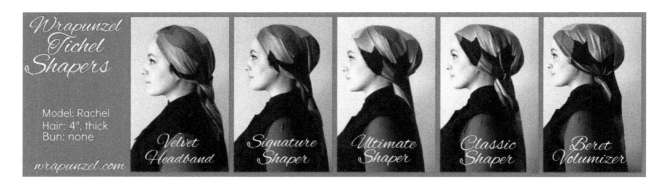

One thing many tichels have in common is that they have volume underneath; sometimes this is from luscious locks, and other times it is because of a Volumiser.

For those going through chemotherapy or with alopecia or who want to add the idea of plenty of hair underneath their headscarf, this little trickster could be a godsend.

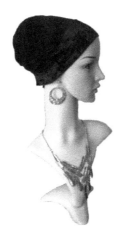
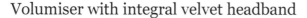
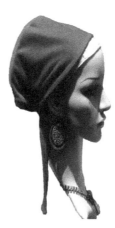

Volumiser with integral velvet headband   Volumiser and separate velvet headband

Ways to Add Volume to Your Head wear

Some women may add volume to their headwrap to appear slimmer, or to enhance the shape of their face. You can become quite inventive! Extra volume beneath the head covering can look amazing! Women with no hair will value more volume as it makes the headscarf sit comfortably and gives the impression of hair underneath.

Padding

With some material (or another rolled up scarf) that serves as a cushion, you can increase the volume of your head wrap, or look for shoulder pads that you can place inside your headwear to work as padding, or a shower scrunch in soft material; put that under the head-wrap to simulate a bun.

A Double Wrap!

If you have a collection of head wraps, take two of your favorites. Wrap with one, then, use another on top. Going at it a second time increases the fullness. Twice the wrap = twice the volume. You could give the first head wrap a twisted bun on top (wrap 17), and then add the second... Out of this world chic! Add chains or necklaces for a Boho look.

Designed Especially for Your Hair

In a store that sells hair accessories, get hold of clips to wrap your long hair into a bun; you can check out the dollar stores for donut sponges to wrap your hair around; with short hair, tie it in a ponytail and put the donut around it.

'Proper' Shapers

If you don't have a great head wrap store near you, 'shapers' can be bought from online stores. Many consist of a velvet headband sewn to a cap with padding to the back. Some even have removable stuffing so that you can change the volume!

Starry Night

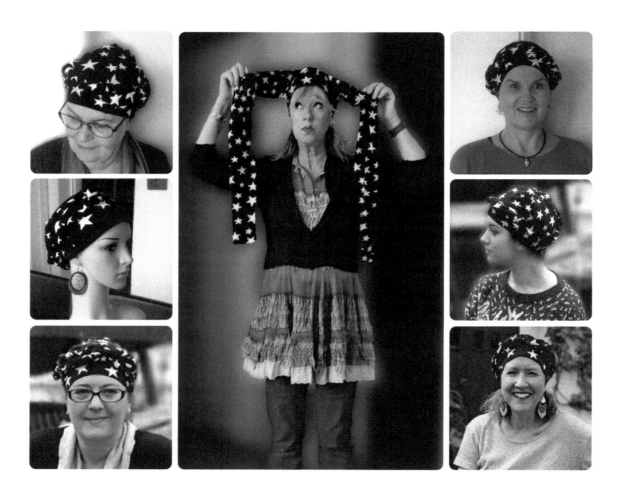

How a small size pair of leggings can become a versatile headwrap that suits every-one.

Starry Night Visual and Written Instructions

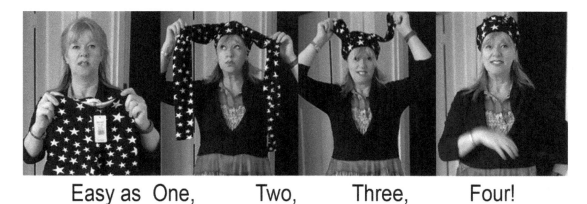

Easy as One,   Two,   Three,   Four!

Take a pair of pre-teen or small adult leggings in a pattern you *love*. Choose ones with a waist band between 1.5 and 4 cm, and yes... if you need to, stick them on your head in the shop to check sizing! The fit should be snug but not too tight.

- Make sure you have the right stretchiness in your leggings (and remember to remove the label before you wear them out!)

- Place them on your head; adjust the forehead to a pleasing height. Cover the top part of the ears and check it is far enough down at the nape of your neck.

- Pull the legs out to the sides, then cross over at the back and bring round to the front. Tie in one knot.

- Then just tuck the ends in; or leave them out and put a second knot in.

Head Wrapping for Free

If the thought of head wrapping is enticing; the thought of free head wraps is even more appealing! So long as you know where to look and what to do, free headscarves are heading your way. As the classic cliché goes, "the best things in life are free"!

Used Clothing

In many cases, size and dimension don't matter; as long as the garment can cover your head, it'll do. So, the question is, can you find an old t-shirt? Jumper? An old pair of jeans? You can visit local charity shops and garage sales, where you'll find scarves going for a song, and maybe some pretty material in the form of a skirt.

Hospital services

If you're suffering from cancer, alopecia, (or any hair loss problem), remember that kindness exists in the form of compassionate people who know the joy a head wrap could bring. If you want a free wrap, ask your specialist if there is such a service in the hospital you attend. Did you know, the elite English fashion designer, Stella McCartney, makes it a mission to design beautiful head wraps for hospitals to hand out free?

All You Need Is Cloth

Not quite free, but cheaper than many scarves…Go to a textile shop, buy your choice of cloth (make sure it's wide enough to be used as a wrap), and let your creative side loose. You can add beads, draw objects, incorporate patches – anything goes! Be resourceful. You can create a bespoke head wrap for barely any cost at all. Look on the *Pinterest* page Kaye Nutman – Headscarves, Headwraps & More for ideas.

Look at the **Pinterest** pages, **Kaye Nutman – Writer**, for *Headscarves, Headwraps & More, Chemo Wraps/Hair loss Wraps, Headwrap Storage Ideas,* and several others relevant to headscarves.

TIPS FOR BETTER HEAD WRAPPING (YouTube)

Head wrapping can be effortless, after you've learned the ropes yourself. If you could use a few tips from the pros, video tutorials are a good way to start: (DISCLAIMER, I cannot guarantee they all will still be there!)

1. Head wrapping without Knots by EyelineHer Videos

- Shows simple Head wrapping tutorial without knots **7.08 minutes**

2. Nine Vintage Head wrapping Tips by Vintagious

- Shows Head wrapping techniques for a vintage look **7.57 minutes**

3. Fifteen Ways to Wear a Head wrap by Love Your Tresses

- Shows quick ways to use a head wrap **9.57 minutes**

4. Double Braid Head wrapping Tutorial by Wrapunzel Ladies

- Shows a double braid Head wrapping tutorial **5.52 minutes**

5. Classic Head wrapping Tutorial by Rivka Malka Perlman

- Shows tips on tying "The Classic" headwrap **3.34 minutes**

6. Head Wrap for Short--Haired Women by Omega Bone

- Head wrapping tips for those with short hair (or without hair) **3 04 minutes**

7. https://www.youtube.com/watch?v=ok4xMtHQMdg

- Turban Tutorial with Liberty London (Dina Tokio) **6min 43seconds**

Complimentary/Analgous Colours

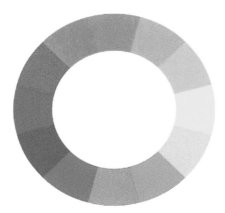

Complementary colours are opposite each other on the colour wheel (e.g. red and green) and create a vibrant look. They work well when you want to stand out.

Analgous colours are often found in nature and match well (e.g. Pale Blue, Blue and Indigo). Choose one for your base colour and the others as accent colours.

Play Matchmaker!

If your outfits are in solid colours, a head wrap in a solid complementary colour rewards you with a contrasting look. If you're wearing a monochromatic dress, you can complement your appearance with something colourful and bright.

With your skin tone in mind, choose a headwrap according to colour. They accentuate your unique characteristics and bring balance to your appearance. Consider picking the families of orange, blue, and red if you have fair skin. These colours can look fabulous in a head scarf. Choose colours wisely.

That Perfect Pattern

Plaid, polka dots, paisley, and floral are among the most common patterns in scarves. Apart from going with the one that you think is the most attractive, focus on a pattern that blends well with your outfit. Try matching your shirt's design, for instance. If you're the outgoing type who is known for her colorful personality, you can incorporate a variety of patterns. Check in the mirror to see that they are not harsh on the eyes; if they're not, then go ahead. Rock that head wrap!

Infinity

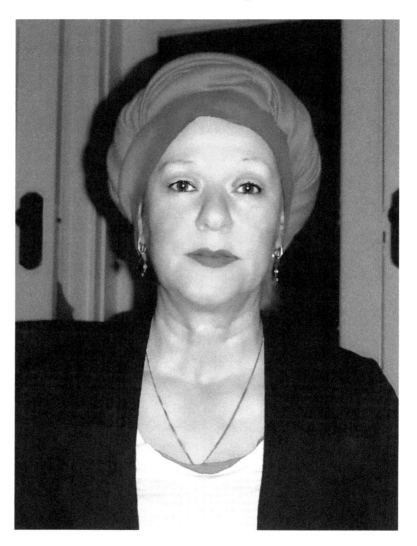

Infinity Visual and Written Instructions

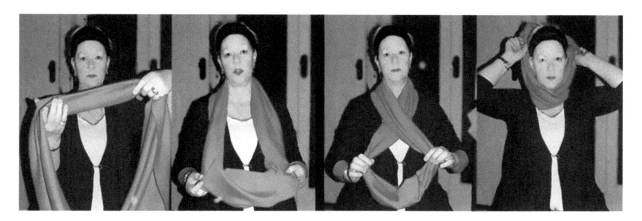

The material I used is known as 'ribbing'. It is used for cuffs and hems on tops. It is available in various loop sizes from haberdashers and large material outlets. Cut to about 60cm width (14"). Of course you can buy infinity scarfs ready-made.

This can be done in well under sixty seconds with a little practice!

- Take your material/infinity scarf

- Place it round your neck

- Give it one twist

- Put the lower edge over your head and let it rest on your neck

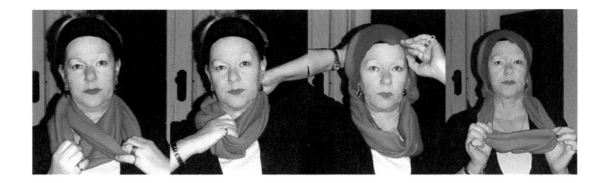

At first you may want to look in the mirror for this part:

- Grip the outer edges and note how it forms a cross over at the front

- Twist the cross over to the back

- Now you have two loops. Place the loop near your throat over your head

- Pull the lower loop out gently and tug to make the head covering snug

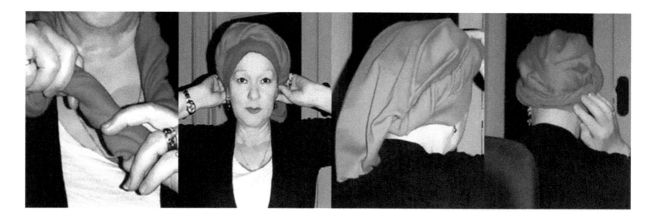

- Twist the loop round and round quite tightly to make a 'rope'

- Pull the rope up over your face to rest just below the crown of your head

- The back now forms a flap; give it one twist, then tuck it in to complete the look

- Hold up a mirror to the back whilst looking in another mirror to check it is neat

Magic Tricks: How to Look Great with Head wrapping

I've said that headwraps can make you look great, but this can be an understatement. Headwraps can make you look *stunning*! A bit of magic is all it takes.

Eyeing Colors Wisely

Let's say you have perfect **blue eyes**. The goal is to bring out the vibrant, rich, and dreamy quality of your eyes; turn to the set of hues that can help you. Most shades of blue can be emphasized beautifully by the colors brown, orange, bronze, and gold, so try a scarf in those colours. Rose, denim, turquoise and mustard could also suit.

For **brown eyes** try eggplant, cornflower blue, green and subtle gold or perhaps copper coloured scarves. Dark brown eyes look spectacular with chocolate brown or mahogany.

Green eyes can look fabulous beneath khaki, blue and gold coverings. Darker colours intensify the eye, so emerald green; aqua, plum and burgundy will make them sparkle.

Hazel eyes reach out for the dark neutral colours of moss green and purple. Maybe a tone of orange, lavender or a rich charcoal colour will make your eyes pop.

Grey eyes can look striking with grey blue or shimmering grey accessories. Don't forget purple and violet, bronze, brown and taupe – or for drama fuchsia, black and silver.

All of the above rely on you choosing a shade that also compliments your skin tone, so look in a mirror and hold the scarf under your chin.

MORE TIPS: WEBSITES TO BROWSE

It's a treat to stumble on websites that feature all sorts of head wrapping tricks - especially if you could use some different suggestions on how to look stunning with your head wear and hair accessories. Along with plenty of tips, among the useful suggestions here are pictures, videos, step-by-step tutorials, and personal experiences. So, if you want to learn how to head wrap better, why not learn it directly from the pros?

- Fifteen Unexpected Ways of Tying a Headwrap by Jiji

  http://blog.jiji.ng/2015/08/how-to-tie-a-head-wrap-15-unexpected-ways/

- Headwraps, Hair Accessories, Hair Styles, And More by My Head Coverings

  https://myheadcoverings.wordpress.com/

- Headwrapping Especially for Cancer Patients by Dana Farber Cancer Institute

  http://www.dana-farber.org/Health-Library/Tips-for-Tying-a-Headscarf.aspx

- Step-by-Step Techniques on Using Various Types of Headwraps by Scarves net

  http://www.scarves.net/how-to-tie-a-scarf/head-scarves

- Cool Discussions about Different Types of Headcovers by Headcovers
  https://www.headcovers.com/

- Just about Every Headwrapping Technique by Andrea Grinberg and the Famous Wrapunzel Ladies   http://wrapunzelblog.com/ See also their YouTube page https://www.youtube.com/channel/UC2XCTY8ZiotLYahaaianj-w

Ten Second Wonder

A fabulous scarf in grey stretch material, with built in bobbles!

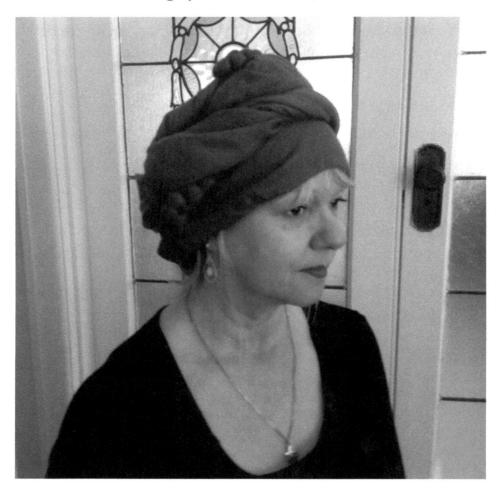

You really can do this in 10 seconds!

Centre on your head, push the ends over your shoulders; tie once at the back

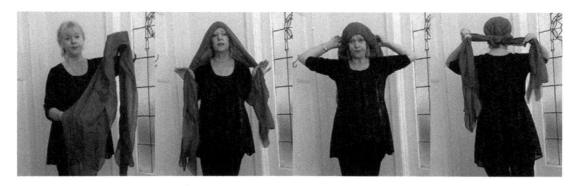

Bring one side over your head, then the other side; overlap and tuck in at the back

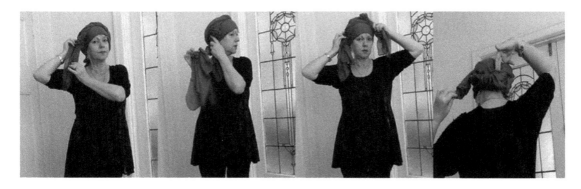

Et Voila!

PINTEREST

My *Favourite* Resource!

You are invited to access my ***'Headscarves, Headwraps and More'*** Pinterest page with 5,000+ pins, featuring videos, illustrations and photographs of a diverse range of headwear, including turbans, cloche hats, hijabs, headbands, recycling ideas... and so much more. Want to see Head wraps on Celebrities? Head wraps in Art? Storage Ideas? Scarves have other uses? Find them here! https://au.pinterest.com/kn23writer/

See how you can match this lipstick to that scarf; how women put on make-up which sets off their head wrap, and wear complementary accessories cleverly.

Maybe you'd like to see what suits someone with a similar shaped face to you; see what can make a round face look thinner or a thin face look rounder... yes, it can be done!

Look at how women carry off their head wrap as a statement, with pride and confidence, and view a history of headwear in this and former centuries.

Click on instructional videos where regular women show how they tie their head wraps - for fashion, modesty, faith, hair loss, and cultural preference – and share their techniques with you

My page is inclusive; every race and nationality, every colour and creed are there to be seen, demonstrating how to look good and feel ultra-confident wearing a head wrap.

All it takes is a little practice and perhaps a little daring!

Don't have a free Pinterest page? Register here: - https://www.pinterest.com/

Then **GO** to my page 'Kaye Nutman' https://au.pinterest.com/kn23writer/

and (please) click **'follow'** Grab a favourite drink and get ready to browse the various categories! ***Have Fun!***

Other Books by Kaye Nutman

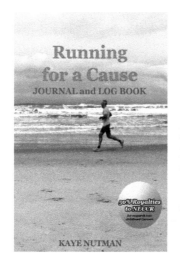 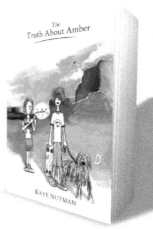

Non Fiction: Running for a Cause   (links to **amazon.com** and **amazon.co.uk**)

http://tinyurl.com/hmmaxtv currently US$9.99 paperback, £5.95 paperback

Children's Fiction: The Truth About Amber   (links to **amazon.com**, **amazon.co.uk** and **amazon.com.au**)

http://tinyurl.com/zcpu6lj currently US$2.87 (eBook) US$8.99 paperback

http://tinyurl.com/z4bd2zy currently £5.20 paperback

http://tinyurl.com/ja7ora2 currently AUS $3.99 (eBook)

(Prices are subject to change)

PLEASE LEAVE A REVIEW wherever you bought this book

Why? Watch this fun video! (Only one minute on YouTube)
https://www.youtube.com/watch?v=Rb0R9zB68CM&feature=em-upload_owner

Then take just 2 minutes to write a review; Only **20 words** or more!

I'll be very grateful, as it will help push the book up there in the rankings, so that it gets seen by more wonderful people like you, who want to learn the secrets to headwrapping.

THANKYOU!

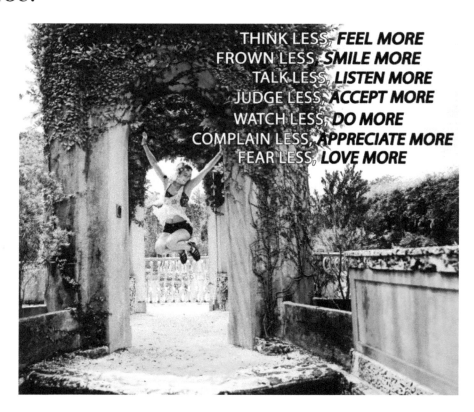

YOUR HEADWRAP PHOTOS

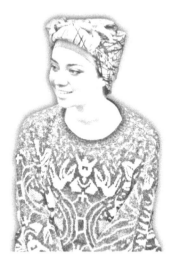

Don't forget to take a Selfie! Why not make your own special *Headscarves, Headwraps & More* photo album? Your style is unique to you!

Email me at anutman@bigpond.net.au or send to me at my web site http://www.kayenutman-writer.com

I'd **love** to see your images!

You can post your favourites on my Facebook page **Kaye Nutman – Author** (please click on 'join').www.facebook.com/groups/360878484067782/

WOULD YOU LIKE A FREE pdf BOOKLET of Headscarf Storage Ideas and Ideas for Other Uses of Headscarves? Then go to www.kayenutman-writer.com

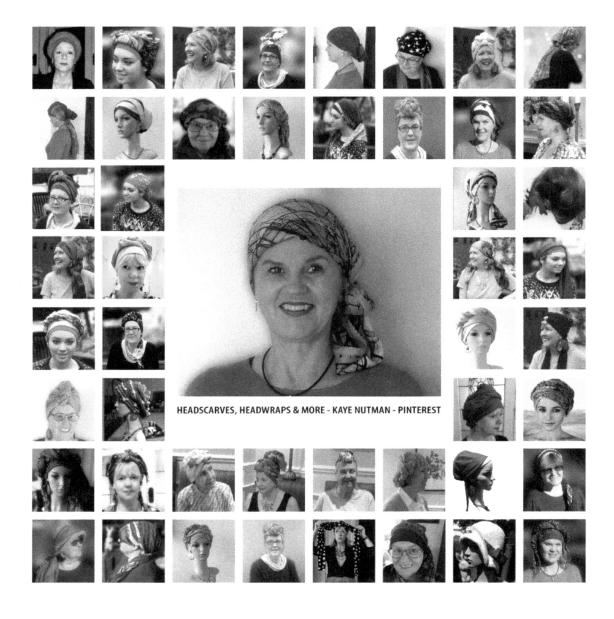

HEADSCARVES, HEADWRAPS & MORE - KAYE NUTMAN - PINTEREST

CPSIA information can be obtained
at www.ICGtesting.com
Printed in the USA
BVHW020716260620
582329BV00004B/162